STROKE RECOVERY PROCEDURES AND PREVENTION

A Step-By-Step Guide to Curing the Serious Illness

DR. JANE E. GALEY

TABLE OF CONTENTS

INTRODUCTION

Amidst a serene suburban community, Mr. Samuel's life took an unforeseen turn. The peace he had experienced for years was disturbed by a stroke, which seemed like an unwanted guest. This book details the incredible adventure of Mr. Samuel, a regular guy up against a fantastic obstacle.

"Stroke Recovery Procedures and Prevention" provides an inspiring story of resiliency and hope in its pages. As we read the narrative, we get to see Mr. Samuel's early hardships, his difficult journey to recovery, and the crucial turning point in his life—when he is introduced to special stroke recovery techniques and prevention.

Readers are encouraged to delve into Mr. Samuel's remarkable metamorphosis via this engrossing story. It's a tale of tenacity, steadfast love, and an innovative healing approach that might change his course in life.

Within these pages, we set out on a trip that goes beyond medical treatments and provides priceless insights into the nature of the human soul. The story of Mr. Samuel is a tribute to the strength of creativity and the limitless possibilities for individual recovery after a transformative experience. Get ready to be motivated as you follow Mr. Samuel's journey from hardship to success in "Stroke Recovery Procedures and Prevention."

CHAPTER 1: Understanding Stroke

A catastrophic medical illness known as a stroke, or "brain attack," is brought on by a breakdown in the blood flow to the brain. It is a medical emergency that has to be attended to and treated right now. It is crucial for both stroke victims and their caretakers to comprehend the several facets of the condition, such as its forms, causes, risk factors, and effects on people. It is also important to prepare for stroke recovery.

Varieties of Strokes

Hemorrhagic and Ischemic strokes are the two primary forms.

Stroke Forms:

Ischemic strokes: Comprise around 87% of all stroke cases and are the most prevalent form. They happen when an artery is blocked by a blood clot or fatty deposit (atherosclerosis), which lowers blood flow to a specific area of the brain. Brain injury may result from the afflicted region receiving insufficient oxygen and nutrients.

Hemorrhagic Stroke: Hemorrhagic strokes are caused by the rupture or leakage of a blood vessel in the brain. As a consequence, there is increased pressure and brain tissue damage due to bleeding into or around the brain. Although less frequent, hemorrhagic strokes are often more severe.

Reasons and Danger Elements

Although there are many contributing factors to stroke, some typical risk factors include:

High blood pressure, often known as hypertension: Because high blood pressure may damage blood vessels and raise the risk of blood clots, it is one of the main causes of strokes.

Smoking: Because tobacco has harmful effects on blood vessels and the cardiovascular system, it greatly raises the risk of stroke.

Diabetes: Uncontrolled diabetes raises the risk of stroke and atherosclerosis.

High cholesterol: High cholesterol may cause plaque to accumulate in the arteries, which can clog them.

An irregular heartbeat, or atrial fibrillation; may result in blood clots forming in the heart that have the potential to travel to the brain and cause a stroke.

Family history: An individual's risk may also be raised by a history of stroke in their family.

Gender and age: Men are more likely than women to have a stroke, and the risk rises with age.

Effects of a Stroke

A person may have significant cognitive, emotional, and physical repercussions after a stroke. The effects of a stroke may vary depending on the degree and location of brain damage and might include:

- Weakness or paralysis on a single limb.
- Aphasia is the inability to speak, interpret, or express language.
- Deficits in cognition and memory.
- Emotional shifts, including anxiety or despair.
- Difficulties with everyday tasks and independence.

Getting Ready for Stroke Rehab

Stroke recovery is a difficult and sometimes drawn-out procedure.

The following are crucial actions to be ready for stroke recovery:

Quick Medical Attention: As soon as stroke symptoms are seen, the most important thing to do is to dial 911 or go for immediate medical assistance. When treating a stroke, time is of the importance.

Rehabilitation: An essential component of stroke healing is rehabilitation. Depending on the requirements of the client, it could include speech, occupational, and physical therapy.

Medication and Preventive Measures: Doctors may give medications to control risk factors including diabetes and high blood pressure. A good diet, consistent exercise, and quitting smoking are all examples of lifestyle modifications that may significantly reduce the risk of strokes in the future.

Support System: It's critical to establish a network of family, friends, and medical professionals for support. As vital as physical healing is emotional support.

Assistive equipment and Adaptations: Using assistive equipment and making adjustments to the living space may be required, depending on the person's condition, to improve independence.

Patience and tenacity: The road to recovery after a stroke may be difficult and drawn out. Rehab may go much more smoothly if one maintains patience, determination, and optimism.

To sum up, knowledge of stroke types, causes, and risk factors is essential for early detection and prevention. Understanding how a stroke may affect a person and their family highlights how crucial it is to get the right medical attention and assistance. Stroke recovery preparation is a complex process that involves medical care, rehabilitation, and a solid support network to enable people to fully restore their quality of life.

CHAPTER 2: The Path Back to Health

After a stroke, a person's life might change drastically and they and their loved ones may face many difficulties. Though difficult, the road to recovery may be characterized by resiliency, optimism, and the possibility of a major improvement in one's quality of life. This thorough manual will examine the crucial elements of stroke rehabilitation, stressing the need of establishing reasonable goals, creating a strong support network, and the significant role that medical evaluation and diagnosis play in the diagnosis and treatment of strokes.

Having Reasonable Expectations

Setting reasonable expectations is the first step toward healing. Understanding that recovering after a stroke is a slow and continuous process is crucial.

The kind and severity of the stroke, the person's general health, and the promptness of medical care are only a few of the many variables that affect the scope and speed of recovery. Patients and their family should be ready for a variety of results, ranging from notable functional increases to relatively moderate advances.

In order to create a customized rehabilitation plan that fits their needs and abilities, patients must collaborate closely with their healthcare team. Medication, lifestyle modifications, and rehabilitation therapy might all be part of this regimen. During this stage, it's crucial to have patience and a positive outlook since reaching recovery milestones might take months or even years.

Putting Up a Support Network

After a stroke, recovery is a team effort. Developing a solid support network is essential to a person's mental and physical health. The support of friends, family, and caregivers is crucial during the healing process. They may provide encouragement when development is sluggish, help with everyday chores, and emotional support.

Online and in-person support groups can foster a feeling of understanding and community. Speaking with others who have overcome comparable obstacles about your experiences, struggles, and victories may be encouraging and comforting. A trustworthy healthcare team that consists of doctors, therapists, and social workers may also provide professional advice and a well-organized recovery plan.

Medical Evaluation and Prognosis

Accurate diagnosis and early medical evaluation are essential for stroke recovery. A stroke is a medical emergency that has to be treated right away. Early detection and treatment may reduce brain damage and increase the likelihood of a full recovery. Stroke symptoms should never be disregarded, including abrupt numbness, disorientation, difficulty speaking or comprehending, excruciating headaches, and difficulty walking.

Once in the hospital, a battery of diagnostic procedures, such as imaging scans such as CT or MRI, aid in determining the nature and extent of the stroke. When choosing the best treatment plans, this knowledge is essential. Hemorrhagic stroke, which results from a burst blood artery, and ischemic stroke, which is caused by a blockage in a blood vessel feeding the brain, are the two main forms of stroke. Different medical methods are needed for each, highlighting the need of a precise diagnosis.

Identification and Diagnosis of Strokes

It literally matters between life and death to recognize a stroke early.

The abbreviation FAST is often used to help recall the symptoms of a stroke:

Face: Make sure the individual is smiling and that no part of their face is sagging.

Arms: Ask the subject to lift both arms, then watch to see whether one sags lower.

Speech: Have them repeat a short sentence. A stroke may be indicated by slurred speech or trouble pronouncing words clearly.

Time: It's critical to contact emergency services right away if any of these symptoms are present. When treating a stroke, time is of the importance.

In summary, the path to recovery from a stroke is a difficult one, but major progress may be made with the correct attitude, a solid support network, and the advice of medical specialists. Crucial stages in the process include knowing the symptoms of a stroke, establishing reasonable expectations, and realizing the value of an early diagnosis. The human spirit is very resilient, as shown by stroke rehabilitation, and each little accomplishment along the road brings one step closer to living a purposeful and happy life again.

CHAPTER 3: Thorough Medical Assessment

A thorough medical assessment is an essential part of the recovery process, particularly for those who have had a stroke. The patient's medical history, present state of health, and the precise effects of the stroke on their physical and mental abilities are all thoroughly assessed during this examination. The objective is to determine the patient's particular requirements and obstacles in order to develop a customized rehabilitation strategy. A variety of tests and assessments, including imaging scans, blood tests, and functional evaluations, are often performed by medical specialists to ascertain the degree of brain injury and the likelihood of recovery.

Facilities and the Rehabilitation Team

Following a stroke, rehabilitation often entails a multidisciplinary team of medical specialists. This team may include medical professionals, neurologists, social workers, occupational therapists, speech therapists, physical therapists, and psychologists. In order to meet the many requirements of stroke survivors, these experts must work together. Rehabilitation centers have the newest tools and resources available, specifically designed to aid in stroke rehabilitation. These establishments provide a secure and encouraging setting for patients to recover their independence.

The Functions of Various Medical Professionals

Doctors and Neurologists: They supervise the medical care of stroke victims, write prescriptions for required drugs, and keep an eye on their general health.

Physical Therapists: Their main goals are to increase a patient's strength, mobility, and coordination by using various exercises and methods.

Occupational Therapists: They assist patients with dressing, cooking, and taking care of themselves by helping them rediscover daily routines and reclaim their independence.

Speech Therapists: They assist patients in regaining their ability to speak and swallow by working with them on these issues.

Social workers and Psychologists: They provide emotional support, guidance, and help adjusting to life after a stroke.

Selecting the Appropriate Rehabilitation Facility

Choosing the appropriate rehabilitation facility is essential to a stroke survivor's healing. Think about things like the location, the healthcare team's experience, the center's specialty in stroke rehabilitation, and the availability of cutting-edge technology. Furthermore, ascertain if the center satisfies the patient's own requirements regarding inpatient vs outpatient therapy and the facilities offered by the establishment.

Quick Post-Stroke Treatment

Interventions must be made at the critical post-stroke phase. It is crucial to recognize the symptoms of a stroke and seek emergency treatment since doing so may reduce harm. Medication to break up blood clots or regulate blood pressure may be part of the first therapy, which may increase the likelihood of recovery. Following the stabilization of the patient's condition, the emphasis of rehabilitation is on restoring lost functions and adjusting to the new obstacles that life provides after a stroke.

In summary, stroke rehabilitation is a varied and intricate procedure that requires a thorough medical examination, a diversified and trained healthcare staff, and a state-of-the-art rehabilitation facility. When choosing a facility, it's critical to comprehend the functions played by various specialists and make an educated decision. Seeking medical assistance as soon as possible may have a substantial influence on a patient's recovery path, since the early post-stroke period is a vital window for intervention. In order to improve their quality of life and navigate the road to recovery, stroke survivors and their families need be proactive and knowledgeable.

CHAPTER 4: Emergency Response

Stroke, commonly referred to as a "brain attack," is a life-threatening medical emergency that needs fast identification, urgent management, and complete follow-up treatment. In this thorough guide, we will discuss the key parts of stroke, from detecting its signs and performing emergency procedures to hospital treatment, drugs, and preventative efforts. Understanding the significance of stroke response and recovery is vital, since strokes may have severe repercussions on an individual's quality of life.

Emergency Response and First Aid

A stroke happens when the blood flow to the brain is disturbed, resulting in brain cell damage. Prompt intervention may be the difference between life and death, as well as between complete recovery and severe repercussions. Here are the important stages in emergency response and first aid:

Recognizing Stroke Symptoms

To react successfully, one must be able to detect the typical indicators of stroke.

Remember the acronym FAST as earlier mentioned:

Face: Check whether one side of the face droops.

Arms: Ask the subject to extend both arms. Does one arm slide downward?

Speech: Is their speech slurred or incoherent?

Time: Time is key; contact 911 immediately if you detect any of these indicators.

Emergency Procedures:

Once you've noticed the signs, don't wait. Call 911 immediately. While waiting for medical treatment, keep the victim quiet and comfortable. Do not offer them any food or drugs. Note the time when the symptoms started, since this information is vital for medical specialists.

Hospital Care and Acute Phase

Upon arriving at the hospital, the individual having a stroke will undergo a battery of tests and examinations to establish the kind of stroke and the best course of treatment.

Hospital treatment in the acute period includes:

Diagnostic Tests: These may include CT scans, MRIs, and blood tests to diagnose the kind and cause of the stroke.

Clot-Busting medicine (Thrombolytic Therapy): If the stroke is caused by a blood clot, physicians may provide medicine such as tissue plasminogen activator (tPA) to break the clot and restore blood flow to the brain.

Mechanical Thrombectomy: For some forms of stroke, a treatment to physically remove the clot may be essential.

Monitoring: Continuous monitoring of vital signs, blood pressure, and neurological conditions to guarantee stability and recovery.

Medications and Treatment

The drugs and therapies for stroke may vary based on the kind of stroke, its severity, and underlying health issues. Common treatments and drugs include:

Antiplatelet Medications: Aspirin and other antiplatelet medicines may be administered to avoid future blood clots.

Anticoagulants: These drugs, including warfarin, minimize the risk of blood clot formation in some forms of stroke.

Blood Pressure Management: Controlling hypertension is vital to avoiding repeated strokes.

Surgery: In certain circumstances, surgery may be necessary to correct aneurysms or arteriovenous malformations that led to the stroke.

Preventing Complications

Recovery from a stroke doesn't stop with acute treatment. Preventing problems and increasing quality of life are continual concerns. These measures are essential:

Rehabilitation: Physical, occupational, and speech therapy are typically necessary for restoring lost abilities and skills.

Medication Management: Ensuring good medication adherence, particularly for diseases like hypertension and diabetes, is crucial to avoiding repeat strokes.

Lifestyle Changes: Adopting a healthy lifestyle that includes a balanced diet, regular exercise, and stress management may dramatically lower the risk of future strokes.

Information and Help: Stroke survivors and their families should seek information and help from healthcare experts and support organizations to deal with the mental and physical obstacles of recovery.

In summary, stroke is a catastrophic medical occurrence that may have life-altering repercussions, but with timely detection, adequate emergency intervention, and extensive medical care, recovery is possible. Equally crucial is the dedication to preventative measures and long-term care to limit the risk of recurrent strokes and maximize the quality of life for survivors. By knowing the full stroke continuum, from detection to rehabilitation, we can work together to tackle this crucial health problem and save lives.

CHAPTER 5: Rehabilitation Phases

Rehabilitation is a necessary procedure that helps people recover and regain their independence after suffering a broad variety of health issues, injuries, or operations. It is a multi-faceted method aimed to enhance one's physical, mental, and emotional well-being. Rehabilitation frequently happens in several stages, each suited to the unique requirements of the person. In this article, we will cover the two basic stages of rehabilitation – acute and subacute rehabilitation – along with the important treatments involved, including physical and occupational therapy, speech and language therapy, and how they address mobility and strength.

Acute Rehabilitation

Physical and Occupational Therapy

Acute rehabilitation is the initial part of the rehabilitation process, generally taking place quickly after a serious health event, such as a stroke, traumatic accident, or major surgery. This phase focuses on stabilizing the patient's medical state, reducing problems, and starting the path towards recovery. Two key treatments performed during this period are physical therapy (PT) and occupational therapy (OT).

Physical Therapy

Physical therapy plays a crucial part in the acute recovery period. It is designed at restoring and increasing the patient's physical function, mobility, and strength. A professional physical therapist performs a comprehensive examination to determine the patient's particular limits and provides a tailored treatment plan. Through exercises, stretches, and diverse methods, they try to develop flexibility, improve muscular strength, enhance balance, and minimize discomfort. The ultimate objective is to assist patients recover the capacity to do everyday tasks and restore independence.

Occupational Therapy

Occupational therapy, closely interwoven with physical therapy, focuses on helping patients recover their independence in everyday life. Occupational therapists examine the patient's capacity to do important activities of daily living, such as dressing, bathing, cooking, and house management. They offer therapies that may include adaptive equipment, assistive technologies, and cognitive methods to help patients overcome physical and cognitive limits. Occupational therapists work closely with patients to develop their confidence and competence in doing activities that are necessary for daily functioning.

Speech and Language Therapy

Speech and language therapy is another crucial component of acute recovery. It is typically applied when persons encounter speech or swallowing challenges due to medical illnesses such as strokes, traumatic brain injuries, or degenerative diseases. Speech and language therapists analyze the patient's speech, language, cognitive, and swallowing skills to build individualized rehabilitation regimens.

Speech Therapy

Speech therapists work with patients to enhance their speech and communication abilities. This involves addressing difficulties including speech articulation, voice quality, and fluency. For patients who have lost the capacity to talk, therapists may employ alternative communication approaches including augmentative and alternative communication (AAC) devices. Ultimately, the objective is to help individuals recover the capacity to express themselves effectively and engage in meaningful interactions.

Language Therapy

Language therapy is aimed to improve difficulties in understanding and utilizing language. Therapists assist with clients to enhance their understanding, expression, and general language abilities. This treatment is especially crucial for people who have undergone strokes or brain injuries that have impacted their linguistic ability. Language therapy may involve activities to increase vocabulary, grammar, and understanding, helping patients to recover their language and communication abilities.

Subacute Rehabilitation

After the acute phase of recovery, some patients may move to subacute rehabilitation. This period is generally a bridge between acute care and a return to a more independent lifestyle. It is particularly advantageous for people who need more time and assistance to attain their ideal degree of recuperation.

Addressing Mobility and Strength

Subacute therapy frequently continues to target mobility and strength. Patients may still be working on increasing physical function, gait, and balance. However, the emphasis switches from quick stabilization to more complete rehabilitation. In this phase, participants participate in specific exercises and treatments that build on the improvement established during acute rehabilitation. This might involve advanced strength training, endurance activities, and functional mobility training to prepare patients for a return to a more independent lifestyle.

In summary, rehabilitation is a multi-dimensional process that involves acute and subacute stages, each addressing distinct needs and objectives. In the acute phase, physical and occupational therapy help persons recover mobility and independence, while speech and language therapy supports in overcoming communication obstacles. The subacute phase builds on these foundations, enabling patients to further develop their strength and mobility. Together, these stages and treatments serve a critical role in helping individuals restore their quality of life and independence following a health setback, accident, or surgery. Rehabilitative specialists work diligently to help patients on their journey to recovery, ensuring that they may restore their sense of self and their position in the world.

CHAPTER 6: Cognitive Rehabilitation

Cognitive rehabilitation is a critical component of stroke recovery, since many survivors exhibit cognitive impairments, such as memory issues, poor attention, and limited problem-solving ability. This rehabilitation focuses on increasing cognitive function via numerous approaches and treatments, including cognitive training, speech therapy, and neuropsychological interventions. The objective is to assist people restore their cognitive abilities and enhance their quality of life. Cognitive rehabilitation not only treats cognitive deficiencies but also adds to a person's general emotional well-being, enhancing their self-esteem and confidence.

Long-Term Rehabilitation

Recovery from stroke is generally a lengthy and grueling process. Long-term rehabilitation is important to address physical, cognitive, and emotional difficulties that may continue for months or even years after the original trauma. This phase of recovery comprises continual physical treatment, occupational therapy, and psychological support. It is crucial for stroke survivors to establish reasonable objectives and have a positive mindset, although improvement may be sluggish and incremental. Long-term rehabilitation is not only about restoring lost skills but also adjusting to new ways of life and learning how to manage chronic symptoms efficiently.

Community Reintegration

Returning to the community is a crucial milestone in stroke rehabilitation. Community reintegration strives to assist survivors reintegrate into society, restore their social relationships, and recover independence. This procedure encompasses several facets, including vocational training, mobility aid, and social reintegration programs. The support of family and friends, as well as the engagement of community groups, is vital in helping stroke survivors rediscover their feeling of belonging and purpose. Community reintegration also highlights the necessity of treating emotional and psychological well-being, since the move from hospitalization to community life may be emotionally demanding.

Managing Persistent Symptoms

Stroke survivors may endure a variety of residual symptoms that need continuous therapy. These symptoms might include muscular weakness, stiffness, discomfort, and weariness. Managing these symptoms is critical for boosting the quality of life and avoiding consequences. Physical therapy and adaptive methods, such as assistive gadgets, may help persons restore their physical function. Medication and medical procedures may also be necessary to control symptoms properly. It is crucial for healthcare practitioners and patients to work together to build a tailored strategy for symptom management, ensuring that the individual's particular requirements are satisfied.

Managing Specific Stroke Challenges

Stroke problems may vary greatly from one individual to another, depending on the location and degree of the brain damage. Some typical obstacles include aphasia (language difficulties), hemiparesis (weakness on one side of the body), and emotional disorders. Effective handling of these distinct difficulties demands focused solutions. For example, speech therapy may assist persons with aphasia improve their communication abilities, while physical therapy and adapted equipment can benefit those with hemiparesis in recovering movement and independence. Additionally, treating emotional abnormalities, such as sadness and anxiety, is vital for general well-being. Psychotherapy and medication may be part of the treatment approach to address these emotional issues successfully.

In summary, stroke recovery is a difficult and diverse process that comprises cognitive therapy, long-term rehabilitation, community reintegration, and the treatment of persisting symptoms and special problems. Each of these components plays a key role in helping stroke patients restore their independence and quality of life. While the path to rehabilitation may be tough, with the correct support, perseverance, and a tailored approach, stroke survivors may overcome their limits and enjoy a satisfying life after stroke. The cooperation of healthcare professionals, family, and community support networks is vital in this attempt, as it develops a holistic and complete approach to stroke recovery and reintegration.

CHAPTER 7: Dealing with Aphasia

Dealing with Aphasia, Speech and Language Rehabilitation, Communication Strategies, Coping with Motor Impairments, and Regaining Mobility and Independence are key parts of rehabilitation for those who have undergone neurological injuries or diseases. These issues might be a consequence of disorders like stroke, traumatic brain damage, or progressive neurodegenerative diseases. This thorough book addresses each of these key components of rehabilitation, giving insights, techniques, and support for both patients and their caregivers.

Aphasia: Reclaiming the Power of Language

Aphasia is a communication disease that impairs an individual's capacity to express and comprehend words. It may be a serious struggle, but with perseverance and the appropriate attitude, success can be accomplished. Speech and language rehabilitation is the cornerstone of aphasia treatment. It incorporates a variety of treatments and approaches, such as speech therapy, language exercises, and assistive communication equipment. Patience and persistence are crucial as people progressively attempt to rebuild their linguistic talents. Family and friends may give vital assistance by participating in treatment sessions and practicing communication methods.

Speech and Language Rehabilitation

Speech and language therapy plays a vital role in helping persons with aphasia recover their capacity to communicate effectively. Therapists work with patients to enhance their speech articulation, language understanding, and expression. Augmentative and alternative communication (AAC) equipment, including communication boards and apps, may enhance communication in the early stages of rehabilitation. Progress might be gradual, but dedication and frequent treatment sessions can lead to considerable progress in language abilities.

Communication Strategies

When coping with aphasia, communication methods are crucial for both people and their communication partners. These tactics include:

a. Simplify and slow down speech: Speaking slowly and using basic, plain language helps boost understanding.

b. Visual aids: Gestures, photos, and textual clues may assist express messages effectively.

c. Encourage patience: Allow additional time for the person with aphasia to answer, avoiding interruptions.

d. Ask yes-no questions: This simplifies replies and eases conversation.

e. Repeat and rephrase: If the person with aphasia is difficult to comprehend, rephrasing and repeating information might be beneficial.

Coping with Motor Impairments

Motor deficits commonly accompany neurological diseases, reducing an individual's ability to move, coordinate, and regulate their body. Physical rehabilitation and occupational therapy are crucial components of the healing process. These treatments attempt to increase mobility, strength, and coordination. Adaptive equipment, such as mobility aids and house modifications, may help persons in recovering independence. Emotional support and encouragement from friends and family are vital as people negotiate the obstacles of dealing with motor limitations.

Regaining Mobility and Independence

Regaining mobility and independence is a long process that comprises various facets:

a. Physical therapy: A systematic program of exercises and procedures meant to increase strength, flexibility, and total mobility.

b. Occupational therapy: Focusing on activities of daily life, occupational treatment helps patients restore the skills essential for independent living.

c. Assistive devices: Wheelchairs, walkers, and mobility aids may give crucial help while striving for independence.

d. Home modifications: Adapting the home environment for accessibility and safety is vital for recovering mobility.

e. Emotional support: The emotional well-being of persons suffering with motor impairments is just as important as their physical recovery. Support groups, therapy, and encouragement from loved ones play a key part in the process.

In summary, dealing with aphasia, speech and language rehabilitation, communication methods, dealing with motor impairments, and recovering mobility and independence are interwoven components of a comprehensive rehabilitation journey. The key is patience, dedication, and a supporting network of professionals and loved ones. With the correct coaching, persons with these issues may make great progress, recovering their capacity to speak effectively and returning their independence. Rehabilitation is a path of hope, perseverance, and eventually, change.

CHAPTER 8: Managing Cognitive and Emotional Challenges

In our fast-paced, technology-driven society, assistive devices and technology have become vital tools for persons battling cognitive and emotional issues, especially those dealing with depression and anxiety. These issues may greatly impair one's quality of life, making it vital to study the role of assistive technologies and technology in controlling and alleviating these disorders. This article goes into the critical interaction between assistive technology, cognitive rehabilitation strategies, and lifestyle and wellness in treating cognitive and emotional difficulties, such as depression and anxiety.

Assistive Devices and Technology

Assistive gadgets and technologies comprise a wide range of products meant to help persons with cognitive and emotional problems. From smartphones with mental health applications to complex wearable gadgets that monitor vital signs, these technologies have made major gains in improving the lives of individuals plagued by depression and anxiety. They give real-time help, giving a number of services, such as mood monitoring, medication reminders, and rapid access to crisis hotlines. Wearable technology, such smartwatches, can track heart rate variability and stress levels, letting users better comprehend their emotional states. Moreover, voice-activated virtual assistants like Siri and Alexa may aid with everyday chores, lowering cognitive load and anxiety-inducing circumstances.

Cognitive Rehabilitation Techniques

Cognitive rehabilitation is an organized strategy to treat persons with cognitive impairments, including memory deficiencies, attention problems, and executive function disorders. Assistive technology plays a vital part in this process. Cognitive rehabilitation programs commonly include technology-driven workouts and treatments to enhance cognitive function. These may include memory training applications, computer-based cognitive exercises, and virtual reality simulations aimed to increase cognitive abilities. These strategies seek to retrain the brain, strengthen cognitive capacities, and lessen the effect of cognitive and emotional problems, eventually leading to greater mental health.

Managing Depression and Anxiety

Depression and anxiety are two of the most widespread mental health conditions globally, and they may profoundly disrupt one's everyday life. Assistive technology provides numerous methods to assist, manage and relieve these issues. Mobile applications for mood monitoring, meditation, and relaxation exercises are easily accessible, permitting users to monitor their emotional well-being and practice self-care. Telehealth systems offer virtual treatment sessions, expanding access to mental health practitioners. Additionally, wearable gadgets may offer early notifications for indicators of anxiety or panic episodes, pushing users to apply self-regulation practices.

Lifestyle and Wellness

Lifestyle and health choices have a dramatic influence on addressing cognitive and emotional difficulties. Integrating assistive technology with wellness activities may promote overall well-being. Individuals may use fitness trackers to monitor physical activity and sleep habits, which can greatly alter mood and cognitive performance. Proper nutrition and dietary management may also be monitored with the use of smartphone applications, ensuring that patients with depression and anxiety are obtaining the essential nutrients to support their mental health. Furthermore, meditation and relaxation applications may assist in stress reduction, making it simpler to maintain a balanced and healthy lifestyle.

In summary, assistive technologies and technology play a key role in managing cognitive and emotional difficulties, including depression and anxiety. They offer essential tools for monitoring, managing, and minimizing the effect of chronic illnesses on persons' lives. Through cognitive rehabilitation strategies and the integration of assistive technology with lifestyle and wellness habits, people may take important strides toward better their quality of life. In an ever-evolving technology world, the potential for these technologies to further enhance mental health and well-being remains bright. It is important for individuals, healthcare professionals, and researchers to continue exploring the possibilities of assistive devices and technology in the context of cognitive and emotional challenges, as they offer a beacon of hope for those seeking to regain control of their lives and mental health.

CHAPTER 9: Nutrition and Diet

Nutrition is the basis upon which stroke survivors may build their recovery. A balanced diet has a critical role in promoting brain function, controlling risk factors, and increasing general well-being. Here are some essential issues for stroke survivors:

Lean Proteins: Incorporating lean forms of protein such as chicken, fish, tofu, and lentils may assist in muscle rebuilding and general recovery.

Fruits and Vegetables: A diet rich in colorful fruits and vegetables contains critical vitamins, minerals, and antioxidants that promote brain function and minimize the chance of repeated strokes.

Whole Grains: Whole grains like brown rice, quinoa, and whole wheat bread deliver sustained energy and enhance heart health.

Healthy Fats: Opt for monounsaturated and polyunsaturated fats found in olive oil, avocados, and almonds, which may help regulate cholesterol levels and decrease inflammation.

Limit Sodium: Reducing sodium consumption may help regulate blood pressure, a substantial risk factor for stroke. Be wary of processed and restaurant meals, which are generally rich in salt.

Eating for Stroke Recovery

After a stroke, some people may suffer swallowing problems or change taste sensations. Adaptations to the diet may be necessary:

Modified Textures: For people with swallowing challenges, meals may need to be pureed or softened for safe intake.

Consult a Speech Therapist: A speech therapist may give help on improving swallowing and speech function.

Nutritional Supplements: Some stroke survivors may need supplements to satisfy their nutritional demands, particularly if they have difficulties consuming a variety of meals.

Special Dietary Considerations

Stroke survivors typically have special dietary issues that should be addressed:

Diabetes Management: If diabetes is a pre-existing disease or a result of the stroke, monitoring blood sugar levels and limiting carbohydrate consumption is critical.

Hypertension Control: High blood pressure is a substantial risk factor for stroke. A diet low in sodium and high in potassium may help regulate hypertension.

Medication Interactions: Some medicines may interact with particular nutrients. Consult with a healthcare practitioner to verify your diet supports your meds.

Physical Activity and Exercise

Physical exercise is a cornerstone of stroke healing, contributing in muscular strength, mobility, and general health. However, exercise regimens should be adjusted to individual requirements, including the degree and kind of stroke.

Exercise for Stroke Survivors

See a Physical Therapist: Before going on an exercise program, it's vital to see a physical therapist who can develop a personalized plan based on your individual requirements and skills.

Gradual Progression: Recovery is a gradual process. Start with easy workouts and progressively raise the intensity as your strength develops.

Balance and Coordination: Stroke patients may face balance and coordination issues. Practicing balancing exercises, such as standing on one foot or walking heel-to-toe, might be advantageous.

Cardiovascular Exercise: Aerobic workouts like walking, swimming, or stationary cycling may assist enhance cardiovascular health and general endurance.

Strength Training: Strength training utilizing resistance bands or modest weights may build muscular strength, which is crucial for regaining independence.

Stretching and Flexibility: Gentle stretching exercises may increase flexibility and minimize the likelihood of contractures and muscular tightness.

In summary, nutrition, and exercise are critical components of stroke rehabilitation. A balanced diet, adapted to individual requirements, may enhance brain function and lower the risk of recurrent strokes. Moreover, a well-structured fitness program, directed by healthcare specialists, may assist in physical and functional rehabilitation.

Stroke survivors should embrace these lifestyle adjustments as chances to reclaim their health and independence, assuring a better future on the road to recovery.

CHAPTER 10: Building an Exercise Routine

In today's fast-paced and frequently stressful environment, addressing psychological and emotional well-being is crucial. Building and keeping an exercise program is a strong tool that may greatly affect different elements of our lives, including mental health, stress management, support and coping techniques, and the quality of life we anticipate for ourselves in the future. This thorough book digs into the deep relationships between exercise and psychological well-being, mindfulness, stress management, and the support and coping methods required to enjoy a fulfilled life.

The Foundations of an Exercise Routine

Establishing an exercise habit is the first step towards increasing psychological and emotional well-being. Regular physical exercise produces endorphins, the body's natural mood lifters, which may help alleviate symptoms of sadness and anxiety. Furthermore, exercise may boost self-esteem, body image, and general confidence, leading to a more optimistic attitude on life.

Psychological and Emotional Well-Being

Engaging in a steady fitness regimen provides several psychological advantages. It helps lower the risk of mood disorders, promotes cognitive function, and boosts self-awareness. Physical exercise develops resilience, making people more suited to manage life's obstacles. In addition, the social features of group exercises or team sports may build a feeling of belonging, further enhancing emotional well-being.

Mindfulness and Stress Management

Exercise may act as a pathway to mindfulness. Engaging in physical exercise allows people to concentrate on the present moment, helping them to disengage from pressures and problems. Mindful exercise practices, such as yoga and tai chi, give the combined advantages of both physical health and mental calm. Regular exercise also decreases the synthesis of stress hormones, eventually leading to improved stress management.

Support and Coping Strategies

One of the most crucial components of creating an exercise program is the support system that frequently comes with it. Group programs, exercise partners, or even virtual fitness networks give important support. These linkages not only make exercise more pleasant but also act as a critical coping method for handling life's ups and downs. Sharing your objectives and experiences with others may give encouragement and emotional support, making it simpler to overcome hurdles.

Future and Quality of Life

The long-term consequences of a fitness habit are typically underestimated. Regular physical exercise may considerably enhance the quality of life as we age. It minimizes the risk of chronic illnesses, boosts mobility, and increases overall lifespan. As we invest in our physical health, we concurrently invest in a future where we may enjoy life to the utmost.

In summary, building an exercise regimen is more than simply a physical undertaking; it's a path toward psychological and emotional well-being, mindfulness, stress management, support and coping methods, and a better future. Regular exercise not only improves your physical health but also feeds your mental and emotional well-being. It empowers you with the resilience and fortitude required to manage life's obstacles and pressures. By surrounding yourself with a caring group, you guarantee that you're never alone on your path. With each step you take and every exercise you complete, you're investing in a greater quality of life, one that promises a brighter future filled with health, pleasure, and joy. So, lace up your shoes, find a regimen that fits you, and start your path toward a better you today. Your body and mind will appreciate you for it.

CHAPTER 11: Preventing Recurrence Experience

A stroke may be a life-altering event that not only affects the person who suffers it but also their loved ones. However, there is hope for individuals who have experienced a stroke to avoid recurrence, enhance their quality of life, and prepare for a better future. In this thorough book, we will discuss several elements of stroke rehabilitation and prevention, from lifestyle modifications and medication to minimizing stroke risk, preparing for the future, addressing long-term care, and comprehending legal concerns, including advance directives.

Preventing Recurrence

Preventing a stroke recurrence is a significant issue for stroke survivors. To do this, it is vital to address risk factors that lead to stroke. Key tactics include:

Medication Management: Following the recommended medication regimen, such as blood thinners or hypertension medicines, is vital to reduce risk factors including high blood pressure and blood clot formation.

Lifestyle Changes: Adopting a heart-healthy lifestyle may dramatically minimize the risk of stroke recurrence. This includes keeping a balanced diet, frequent exercise, smoking cessation, and minimizing alcohol use.

Regular Check-Ups: Consistent follow-up with healthcare experts for check-ups and monitoring of risk factors is crucial. Any changes in blood pressure, cholesterol levels, or medication modifications should be quickly addressed.

Lifestyle Changes and Medication

Lifestyle adjustments and drugs play a significant role in stroke healing and prevention. Here's a deeper look at each aspect:

Lifestyle Changes

a. Diet: A diet rich in fruits, vegetables, whole grains, and lean meats may help decrease cholesterol and blood pressure, decreasing the risk of another stroke.

b. Exercise: Regular physical exercise not only improves cardiovascular health but also helps in weight control and overall well-being.

c. Smoking Cessation: Quitting smoking decreases the risk of blood clots and helps enhance lung and heart health.

d. Alcohol: Limiting alcohol intake may decrease blood pressure and minimize the likelihood of atrial fibrillation, a recognized risk factor for stroke.

Medication

a. Blood Thinners: Anticoagulants and antiplatelet medicines may help prevent blood clots that may contribute to a stroke.

b. Hypertension Medications: Medications to control high blood pressure are commonly recommended to lower the risk of recurrent strokes.

c. Cholesterol Medications: Statins may help decrease cholesterol levels, lowering the risk of arterial blockages.

Reducing Stroke Risk

In addition to medication and lifestyle adjustments, stroke risk may be further decreased by concentrating on other critical areas of post-stroke life:

Atrial Fibrillation Management: For patients with atrial fibrillation, controlling this illness is critical to avoid blood clots and strokes.

Diabetes Control: Proper control of diabetes via medication, food, and exercise is vital in decreasing stroke risk.

Weight Management: Achieving and maintaining a healthy weight is crucial to controlling risk factors such high blood pressure, diabetes, and cholesterol levels.

Stress Reduction: Effective stress management practices, such as mindfulness and relaxation exercises, may help minimize the risk of stroke.

Planning for the Future: Planning for the future after a stroke is vital for having a good quality of life.

Key aspects Include

Rehabilitation: Stroke patients may benefit from physical, occupational, and speech therapy to restore independence and improve communication abilities.

Emotional Support: Seeking emotional support via therapy or support groups may assist manage post-stroke sadness, anxiety, or emotional issues.

Social Engagement: Staying connected with friends and family, engaging in social events, and pursuing hobbies may boost the overall well-being.

Financial Planning: Addressing financial concerns and gaining insurance coverage is vital to support continuing medical bills and secure a pleasant future.

Long-Term Care and Legal Matters

As stroke survivors mature, they may need long-term care. Addressing legal concerns and prior directives is crucial for ensuring their desires are respected:

Long-Term Care choices: Explore long-term care choices, such as home health care, assisted living, or nursing homes, depending on individual requirements and resources.

Legal Matters: Consult with an attorney to draft crucial legal papers, including a will, power of attorney, and healthcare proxy, to explain your wishes in case of incapacity.

Advance Directives

Advance directives are legal papers that transmit a person's healthcare desires when they are unable to make choices. They often include:

Living Will: Specifies the medical treatments and interventions you do or do not want in particular conditions.

Health Care Proxy: Designates a trustworthy person to make healthcare choices on your behalf if you are unable to do so.

Do-Not-Resuscitate (DNR) Order: Informs medical practitioners not to conduct cardiopulmonary resuscitation (CPR) in particular conditions.

In summary, preventing stroke recurrence, increasing quality of life, preparing for the future, and addressing long-term care and legal problems are critical parts of stroke rehabilitation and prevention. By following these instructions and working closely with healthcare providers and support networks, stroke survivors may lead satisfying lives and keep their independence while minimizing the risk of future stroke. Taking preemptive actions is crucial to ensure a better and more secure future following a stroke.

CONCLUSION

In conclusion, "Stroke Recovery Procedures and Prevention" is a source of information and a light of hope for everybody affected by stroke. This book is a lifeline, not just a reference. Readers will discover within its pages not only the medical details surrounding the recovery from stroke, but also personal accounts that serve as a constant reminder of the spirit of perseverance.

We are constantly reminded throughout the book that recovering after a stroke involves not just physical healing but also a significant emotional and mental metamorphosis. It emphasizes the value of love, tolerance, and tenacity and calls on the strength of the person as well as their network of supporters. "Stroke Recovery Procedures and Prevention" is a tribute to the human spirit's tenacity and the amazing advancements made possible by willpower and the appropriate direction. It gives readers the skills to take control of their rehabilitation and fosters a feeling of empowerment by motivating them to do so.

Ultimately, this book serves as more than simply a guide—rather, it is a compass that points the way to a more promising future. It serves as a reminder that a stroke is just one chapter in a person's life story and that the true tale is about overcoming hardship and rising above it. "Stroke Recovery Procedures and Prevention" is a lifesaver for anybody looking for solace and hope after a stroke. It is more than simply a book.

Dear valued readers,

We'd like to convey our heartfelt gratitude for choosing to read our book and investing time in it. We appreciate your unwavering support and insightful suggestions. As writers, we are committed to creating engaging content, and your assistance in providing an impartial evaluation would be much appreciated. Your feedback is valuable not only to us, but also to future readers who rely on knowledgeable views when selecting their next book. Whether you felt our book was wonderful or had problems, your feedback serves as an ongoing source of inspiration for us to develop stories that really engage you.

We'd appreciate it if you could take a few moments to leave your feedback on Amazon. Your comment has the potential to have a significant impact on our book's success and reach, helping it to reach a broader audience. Your review does not have to be extensive or difficult; just sharing your thoughts, stressing items that resonated with you, or addressing key issues would be very appreciated. We'd like to thank you one again for being a part of our literary journey. We rely on your continuing support and engagement. We are excited to read your assessments and collaborate with you.

Best wishes!

RECOVERY CHECK-UP JOURNAL

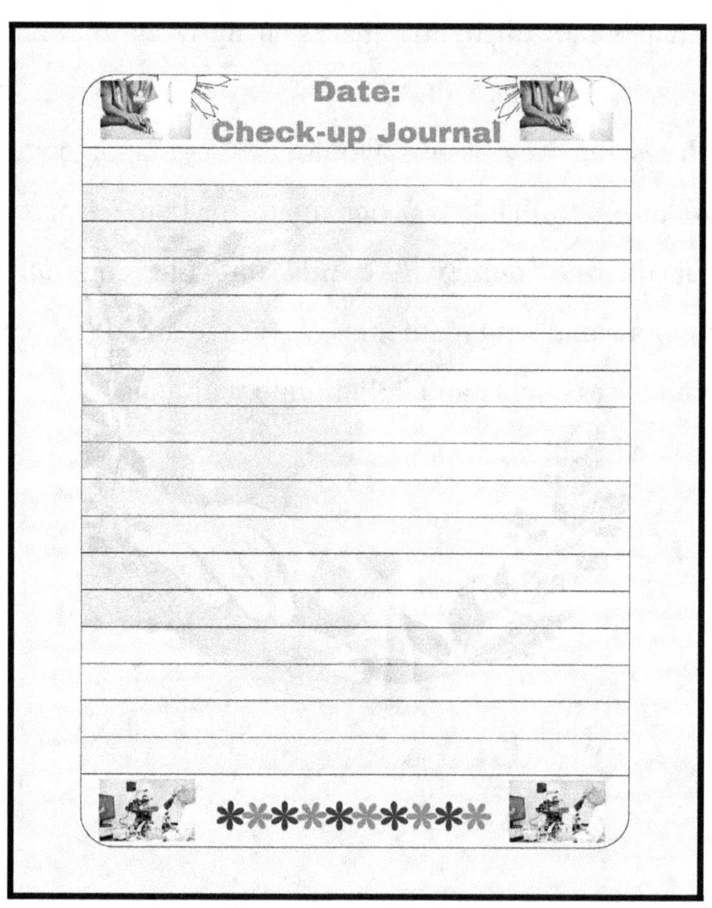

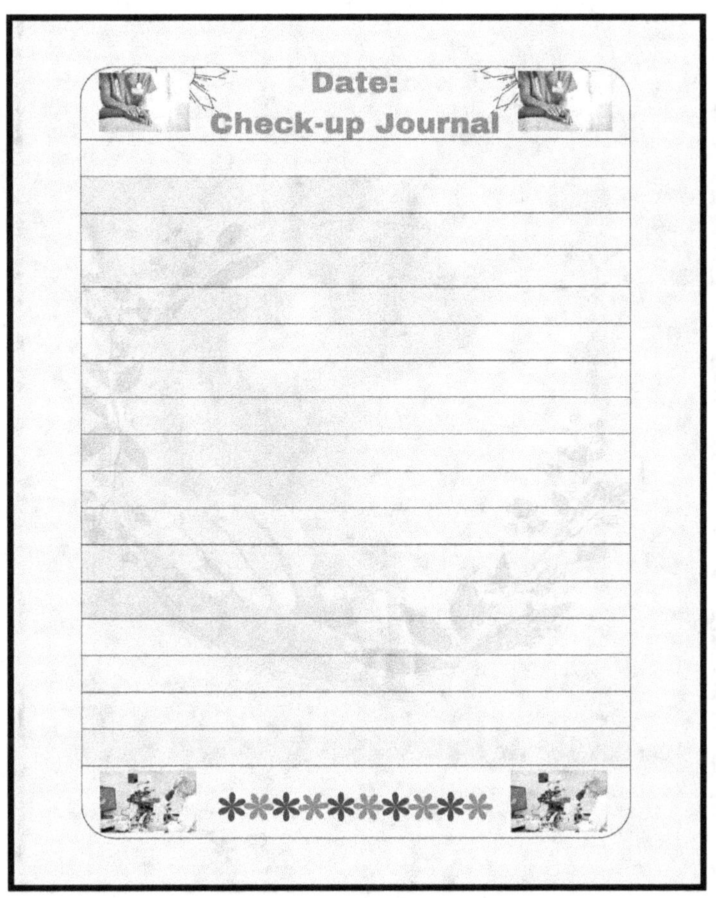

Date:
Check-up Journal
****

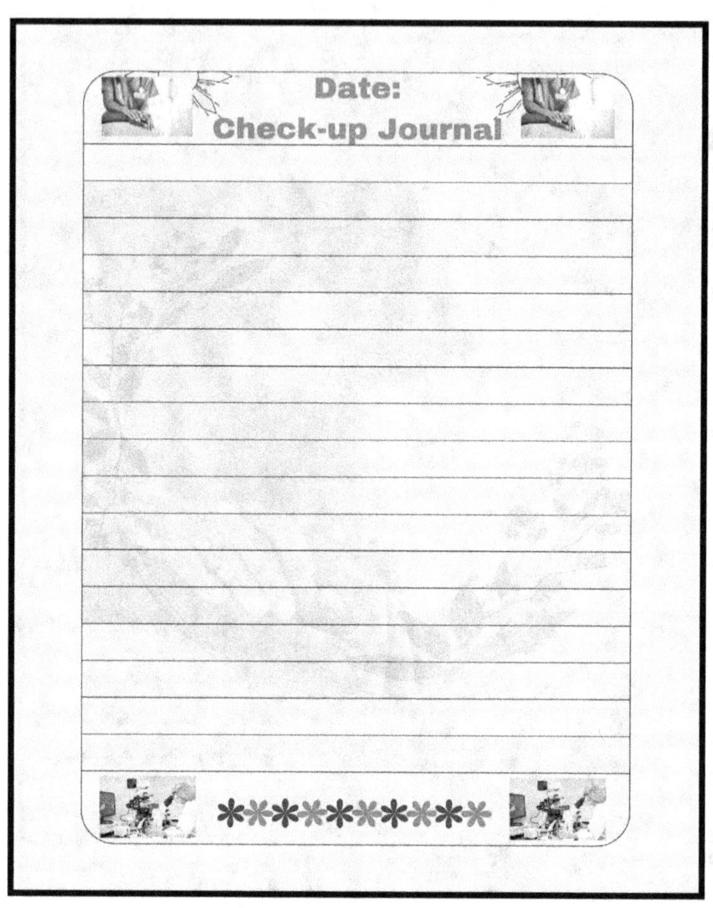

Date:
Check-up Journal

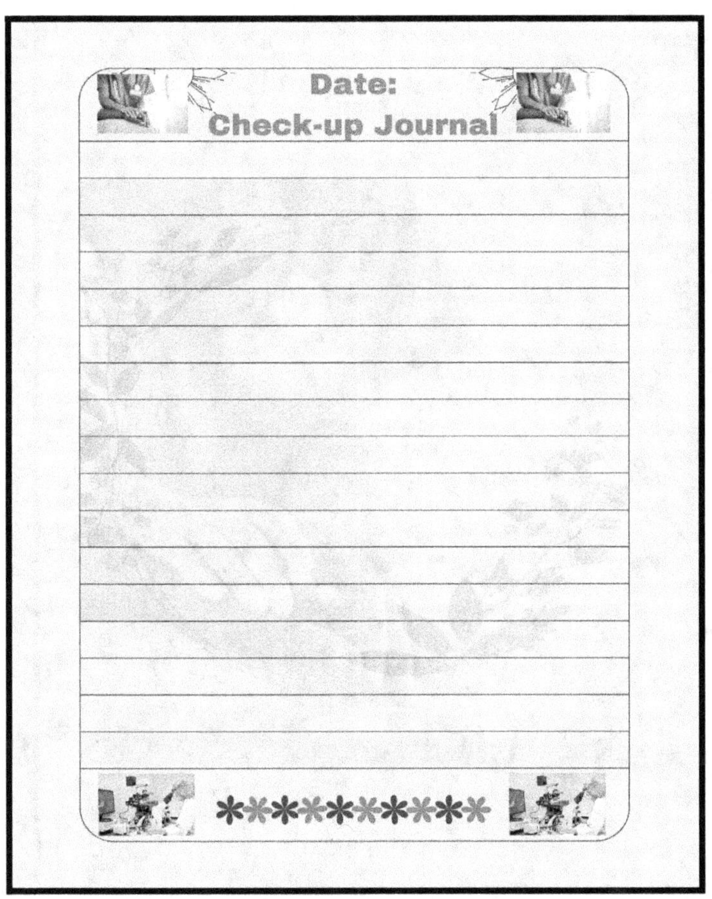

Date:
Check-up Journal
****

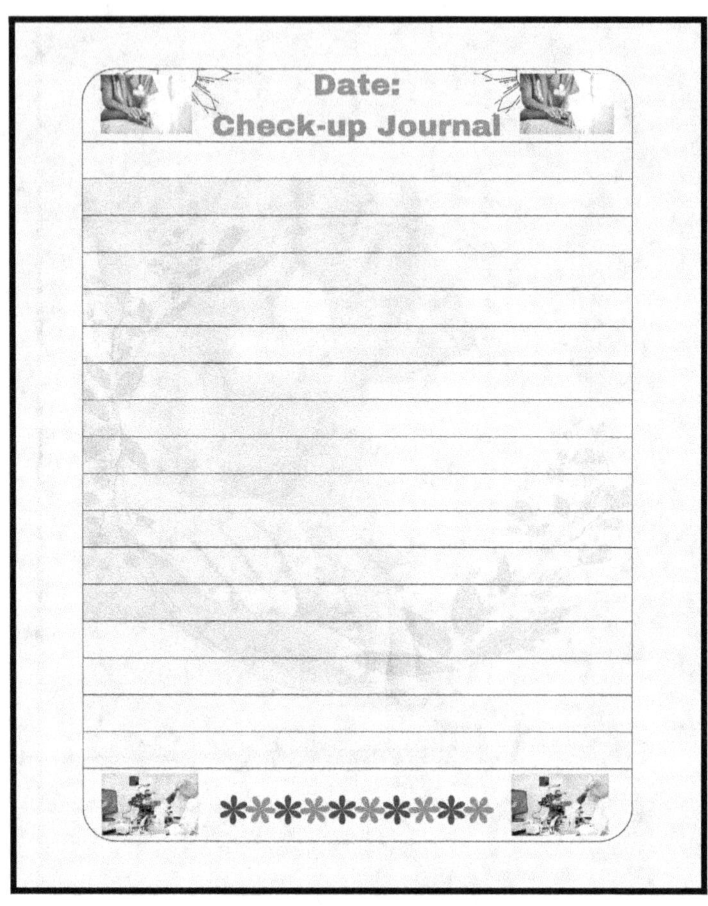

Date:
Check-up Journal

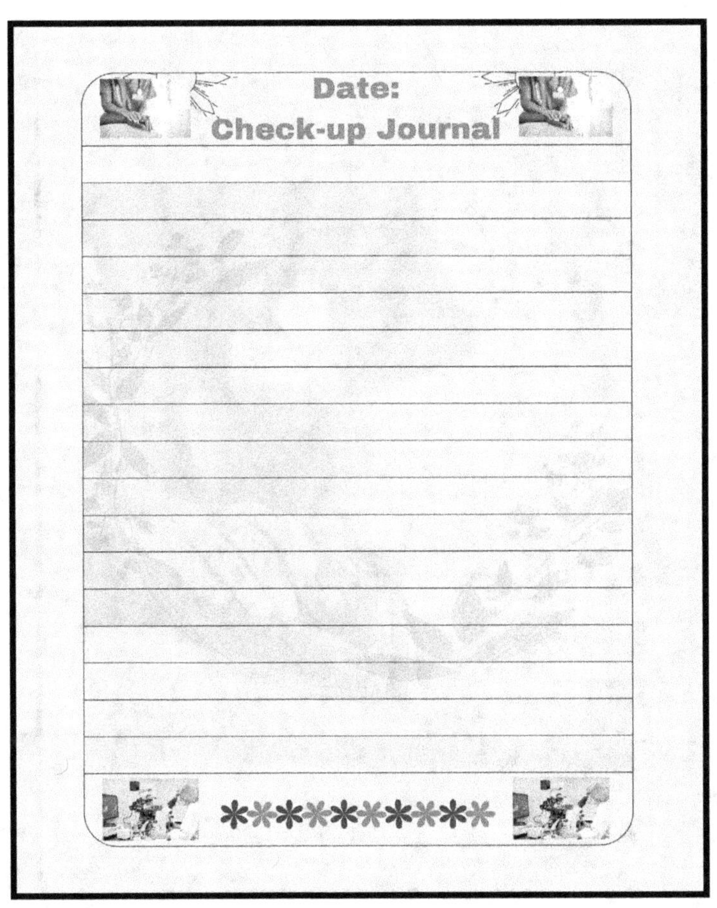
Date:
Check-up Journal
****

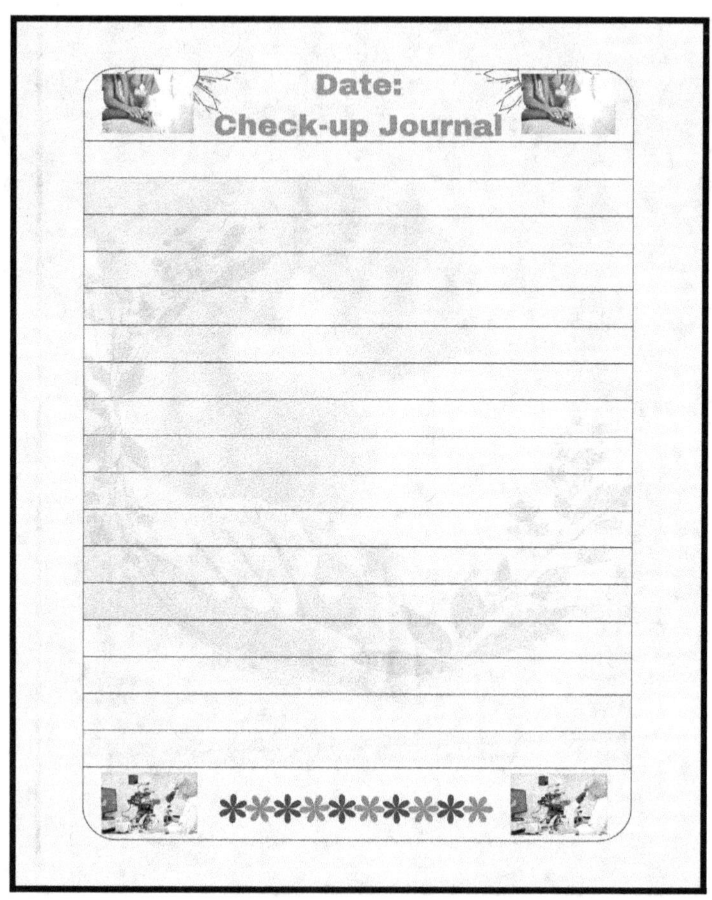

Date:
Check-up Journal

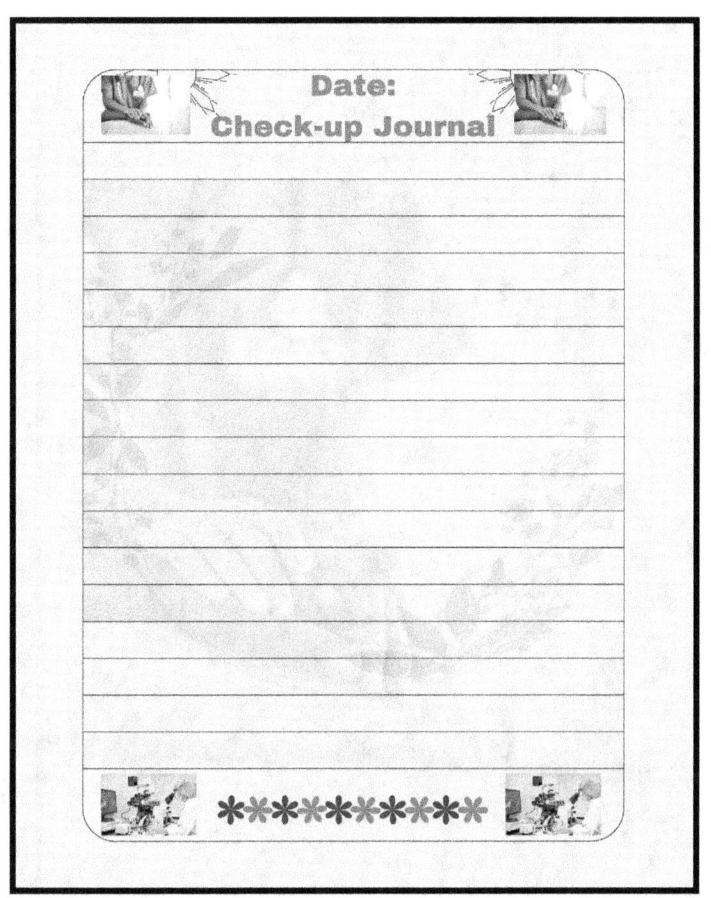
Date:
Check-up Journal
****

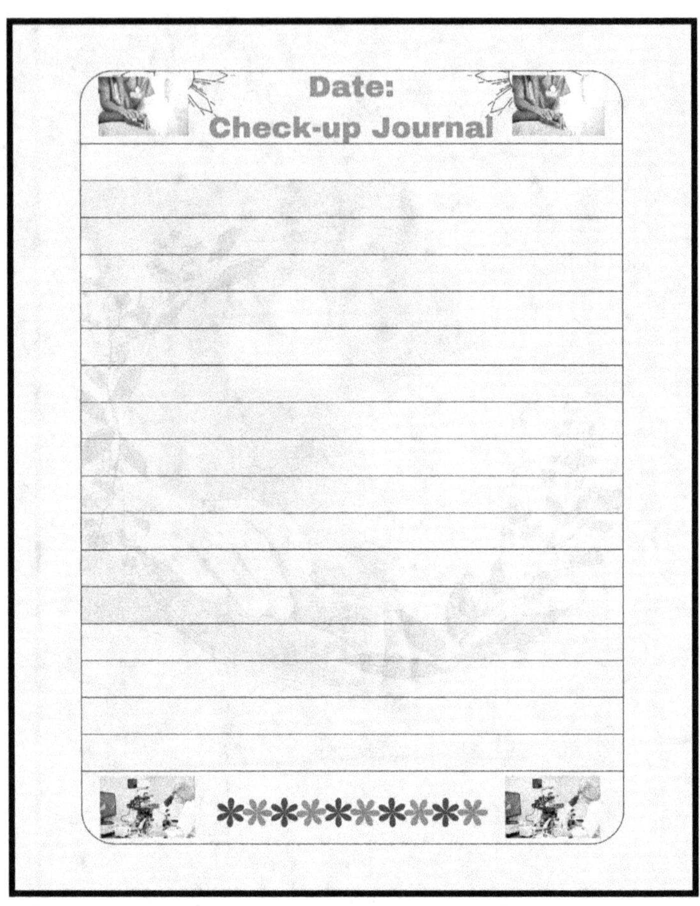
Date:
Check-up Journal
****

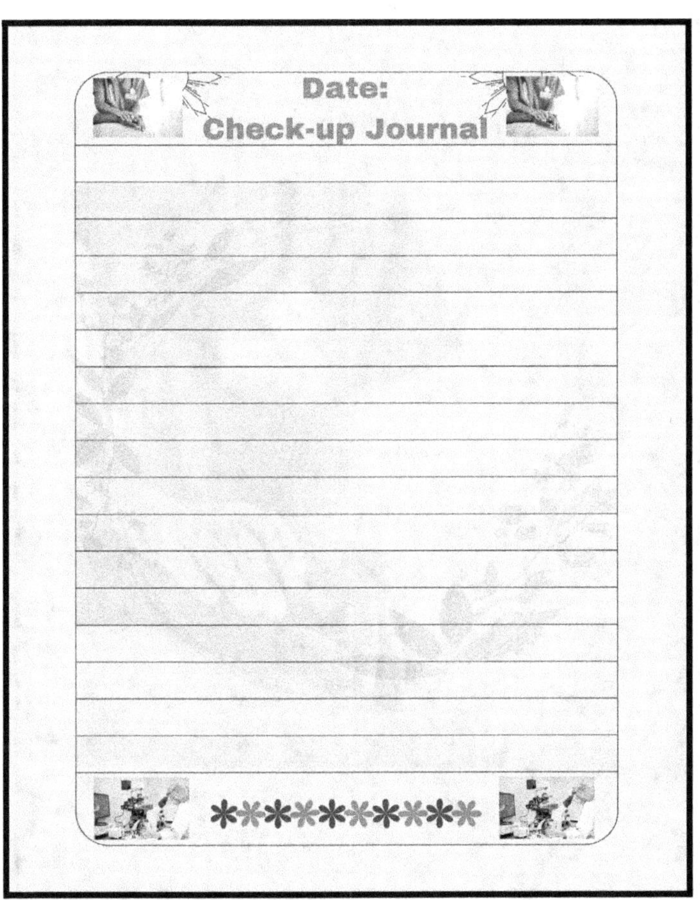

Date:
Check-up Journal
****

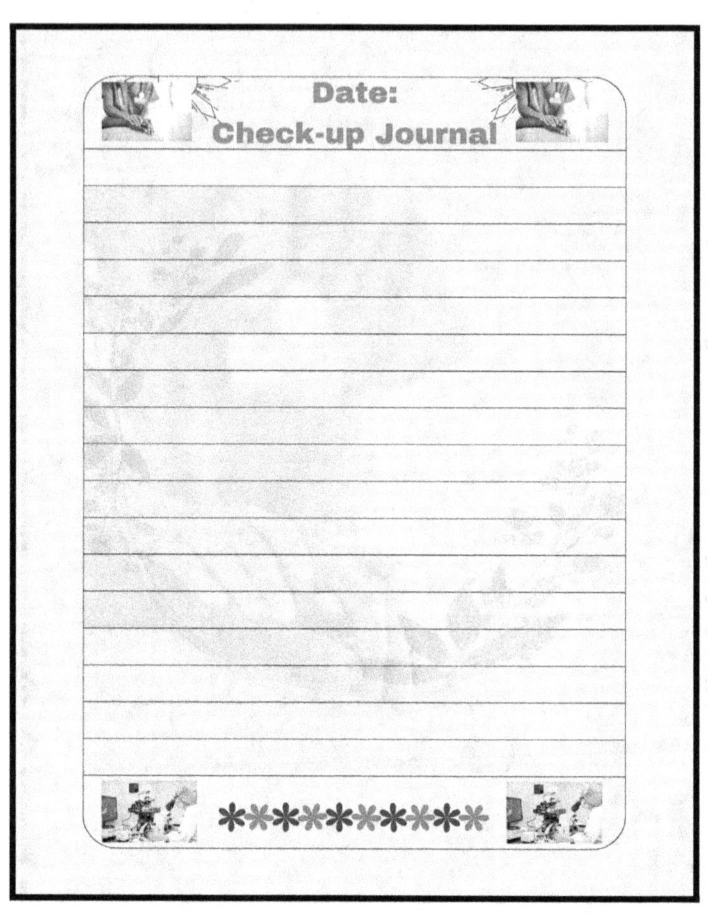
Date:
Check-up Journal
****

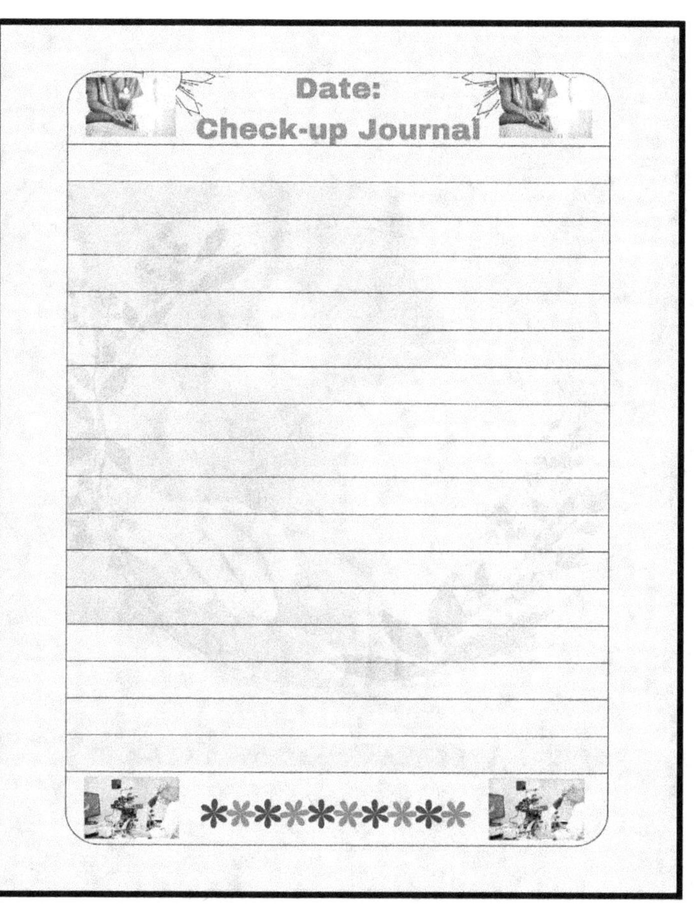
Date:
Check-up Journal
****

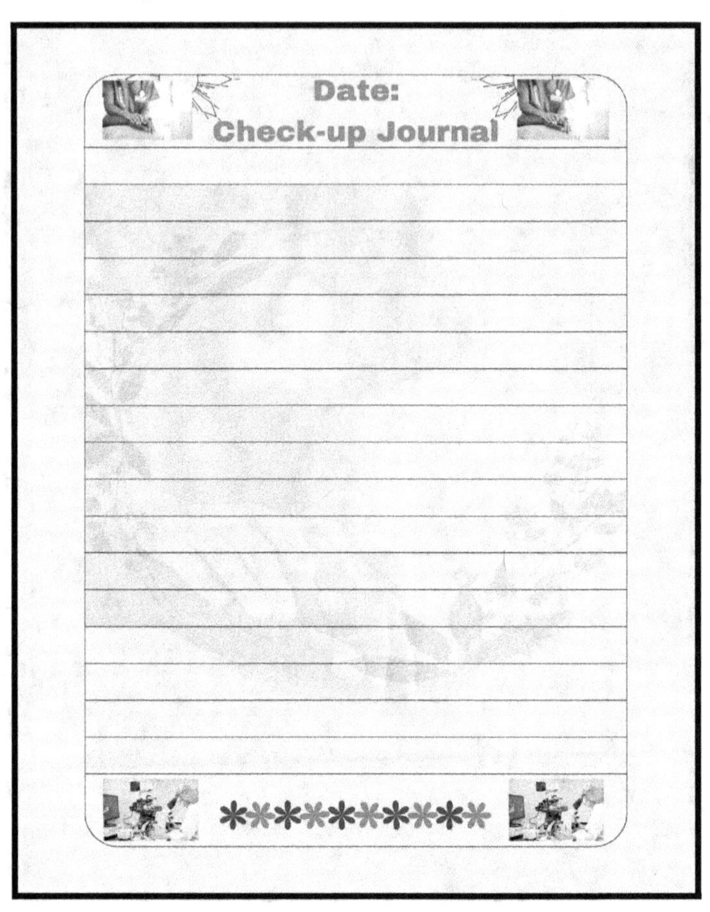

Date:
Check-up Journal
****

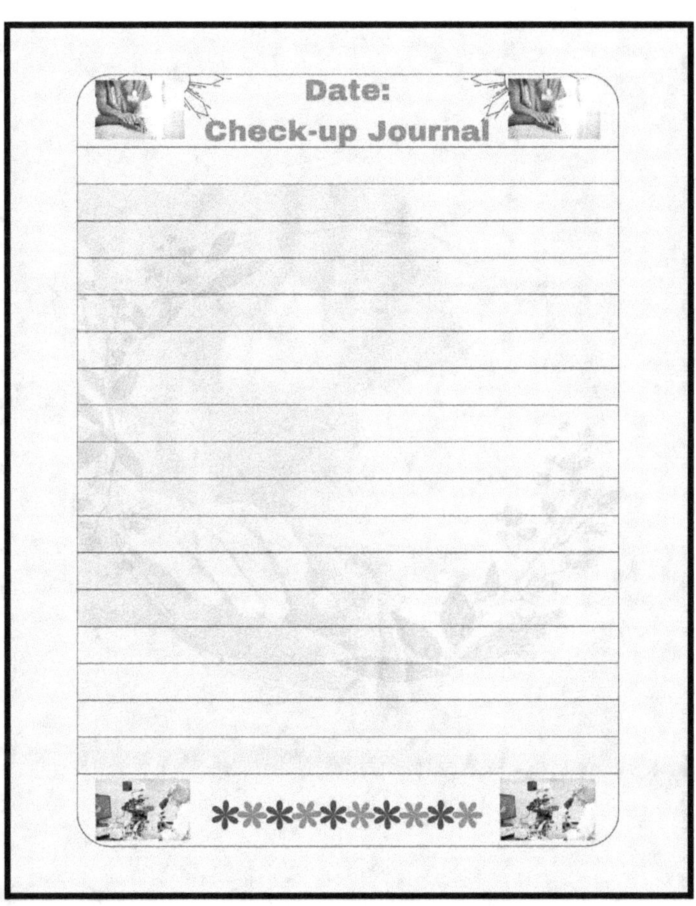
Date:
Check-up Journal
****

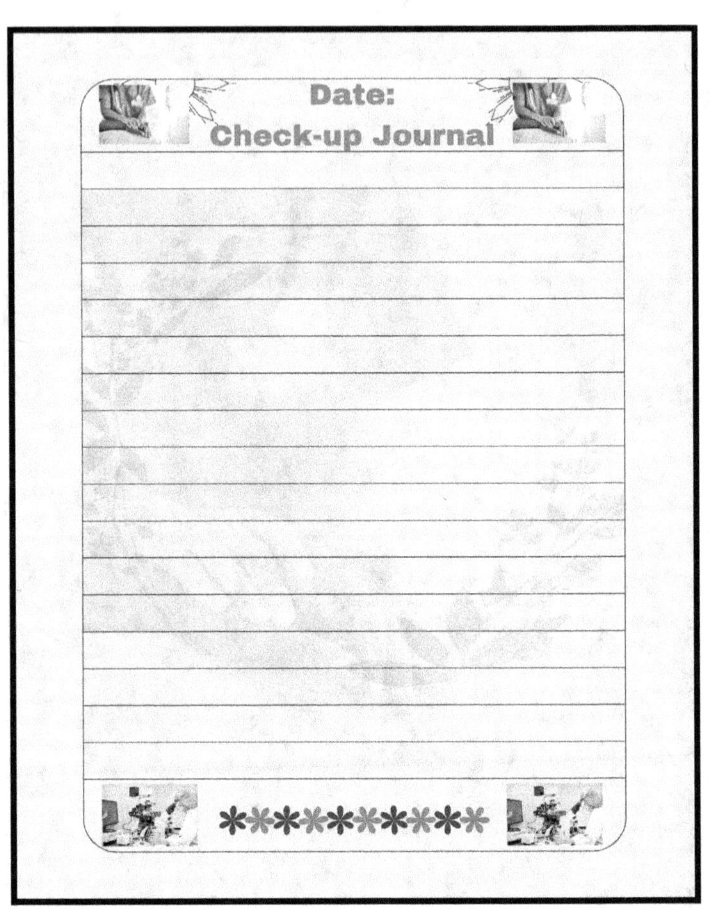

Date:
Check-up Journal

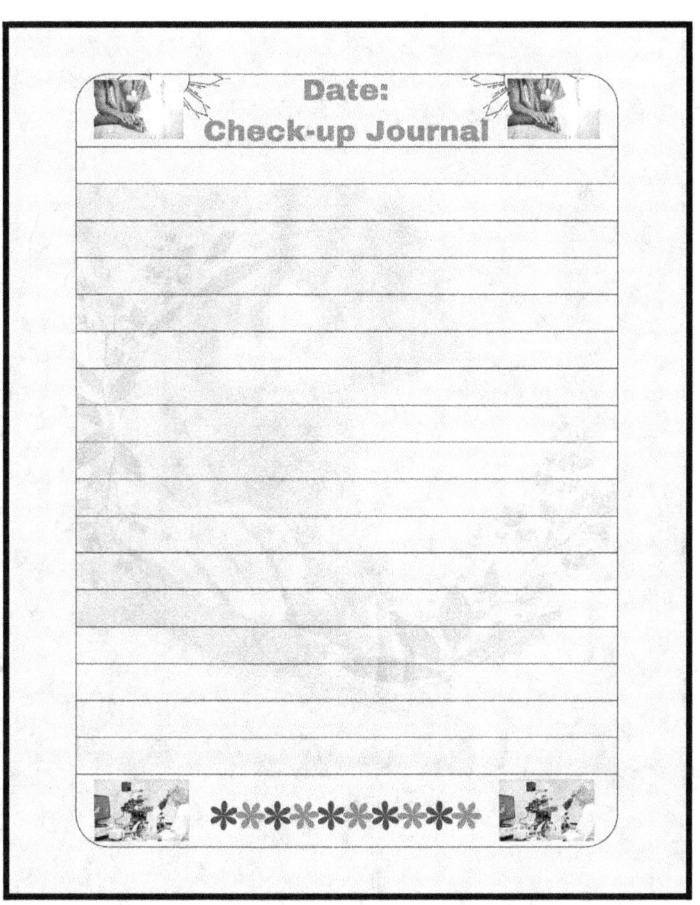

Date:
Check-up Journal

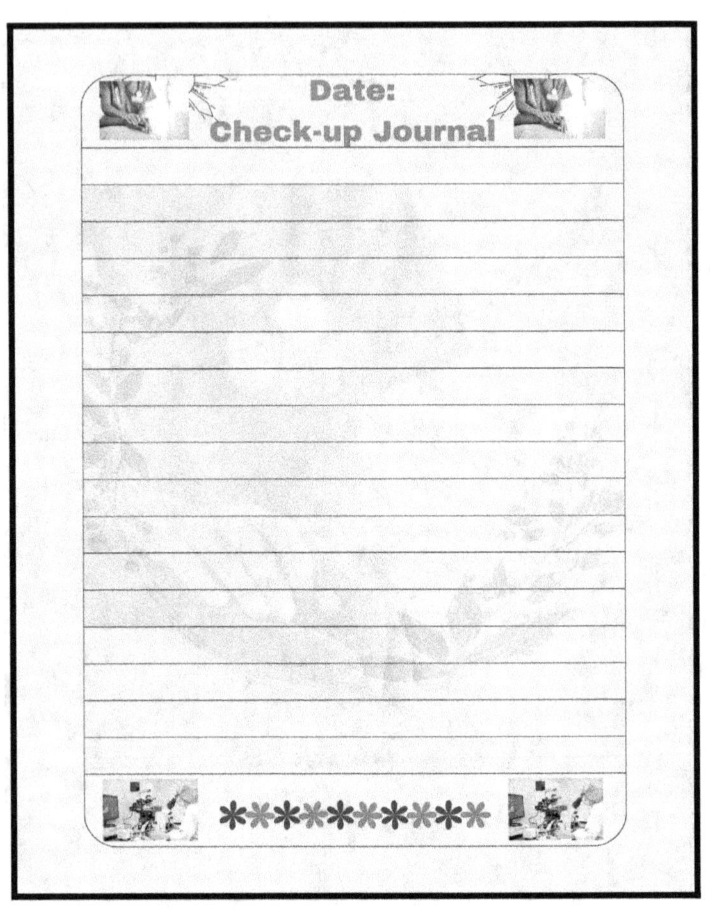

Date:
Check-up Journal
****

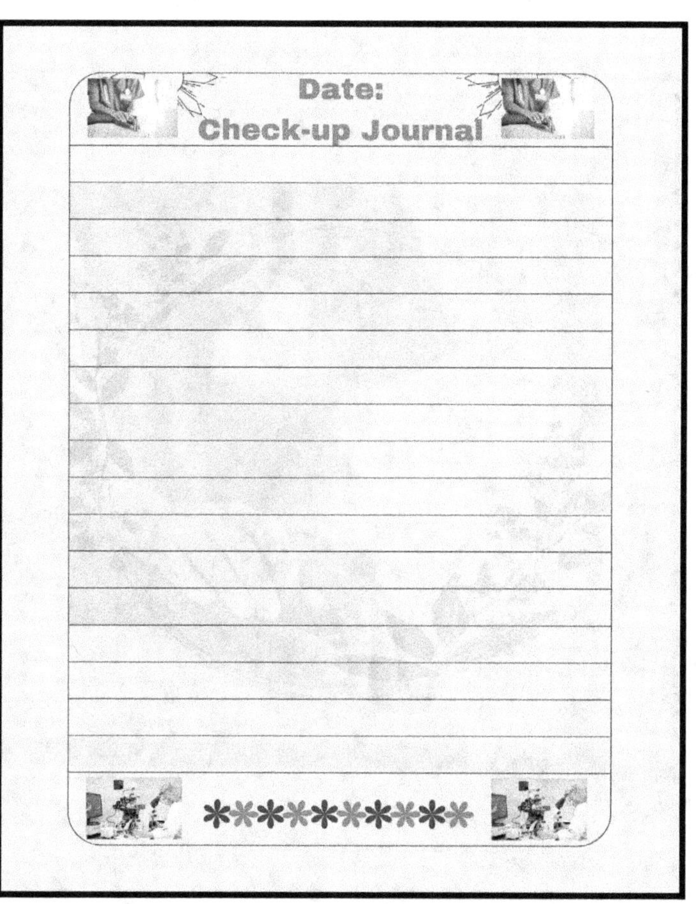

Date:
Check-up Journal

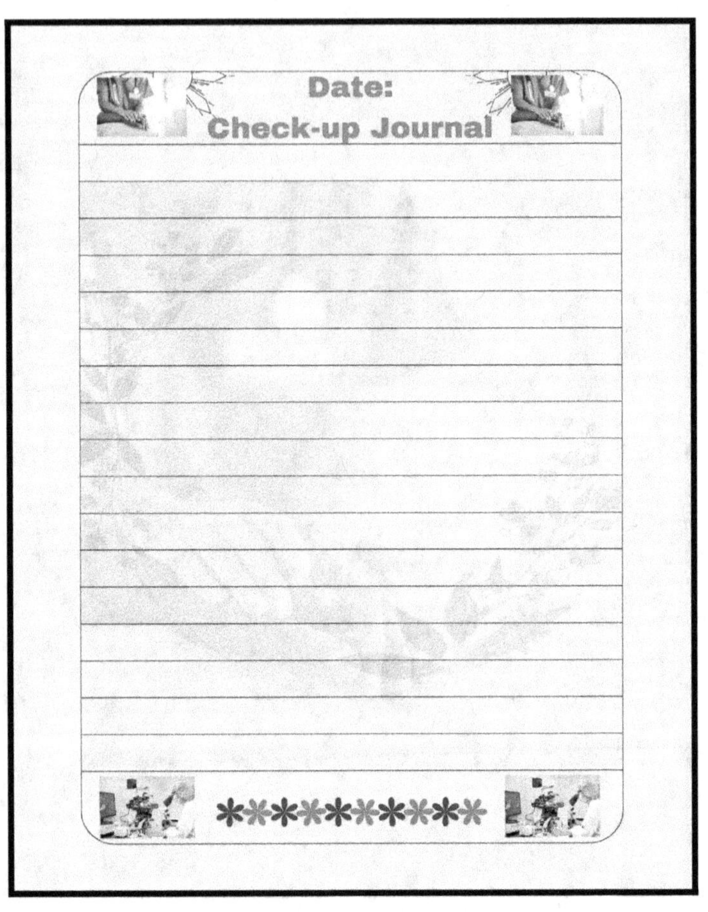

Date:
Check-up Journal
****

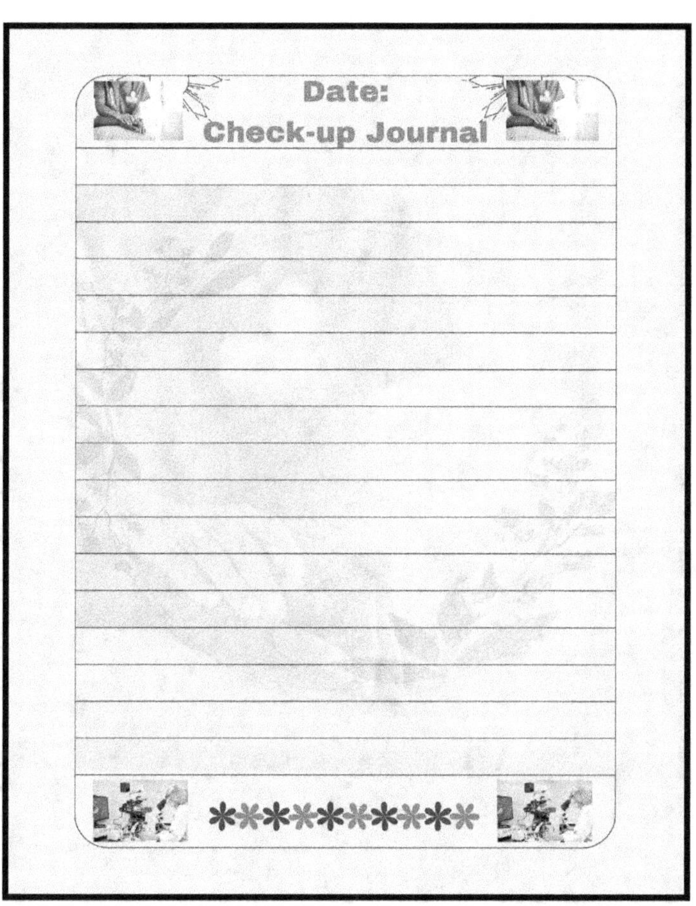

Date:
Check-up Journal

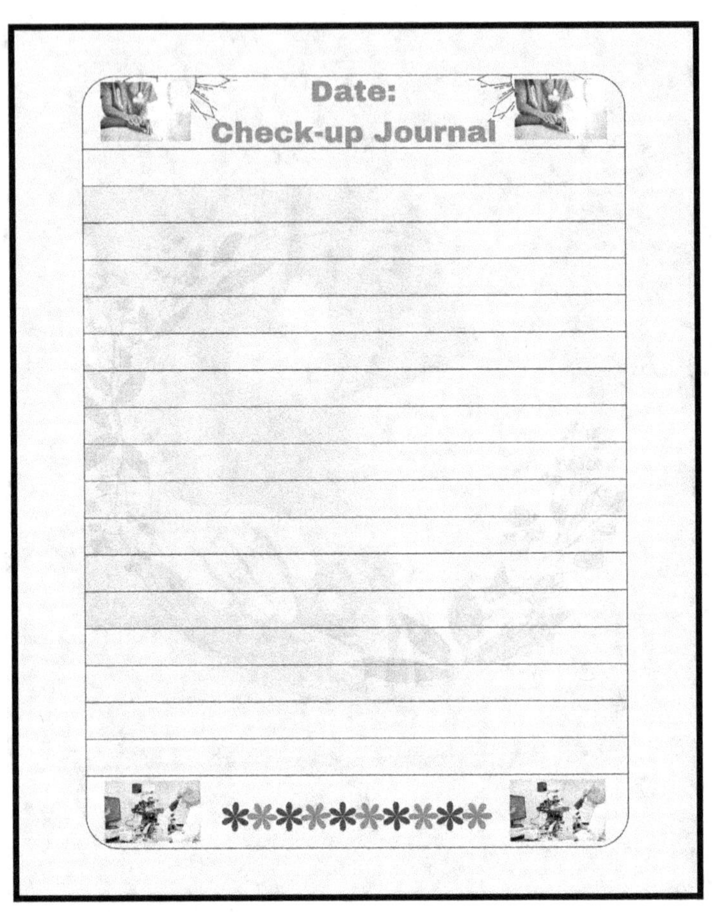
Date:
Check-up Journal
****

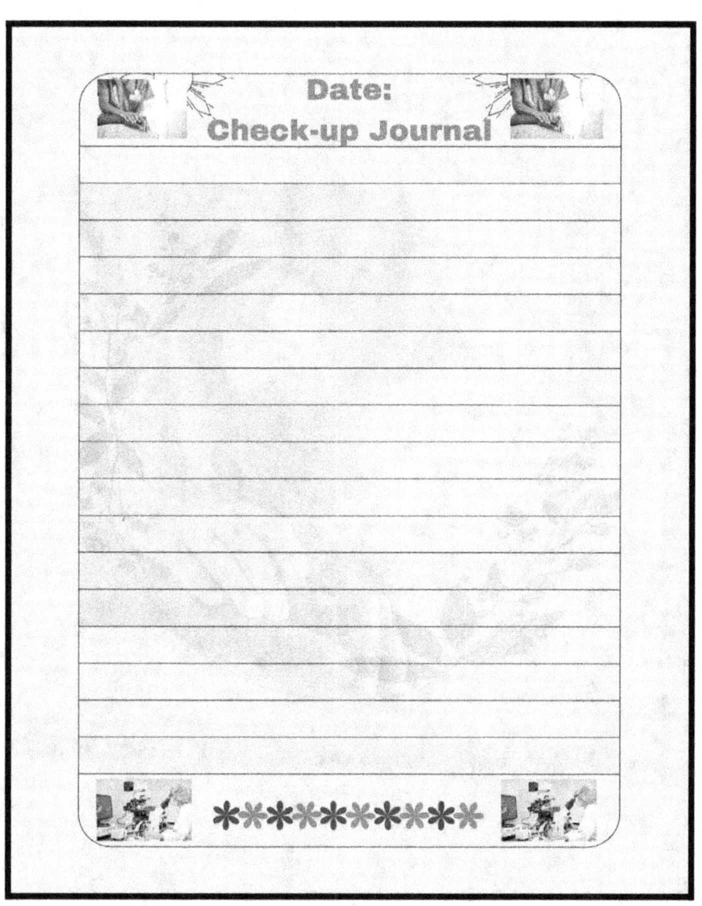

Date:
Check-up Journal

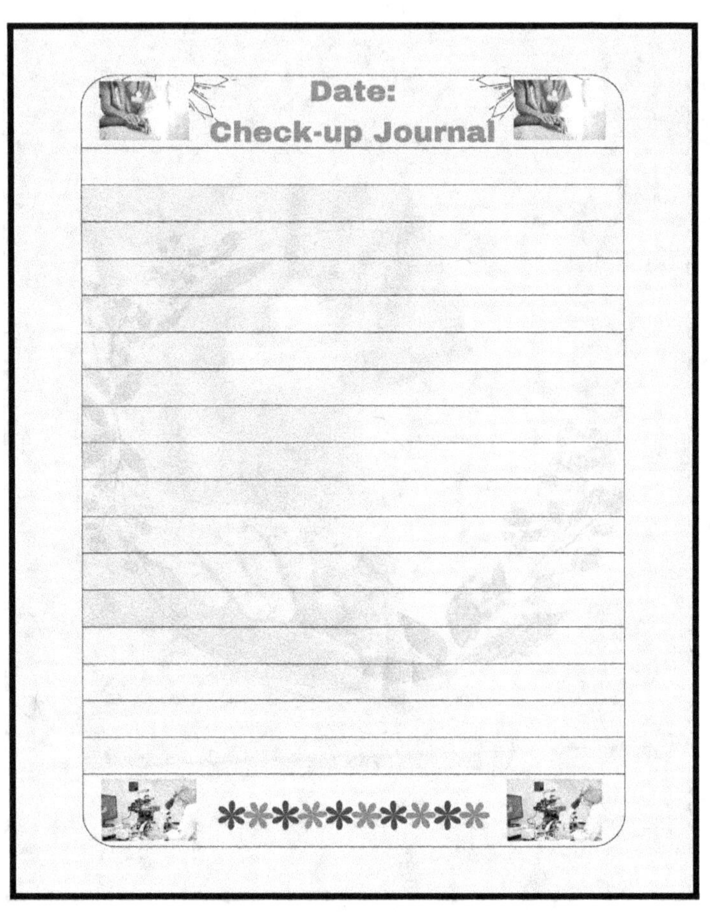

Date:
Check-up Journal
****

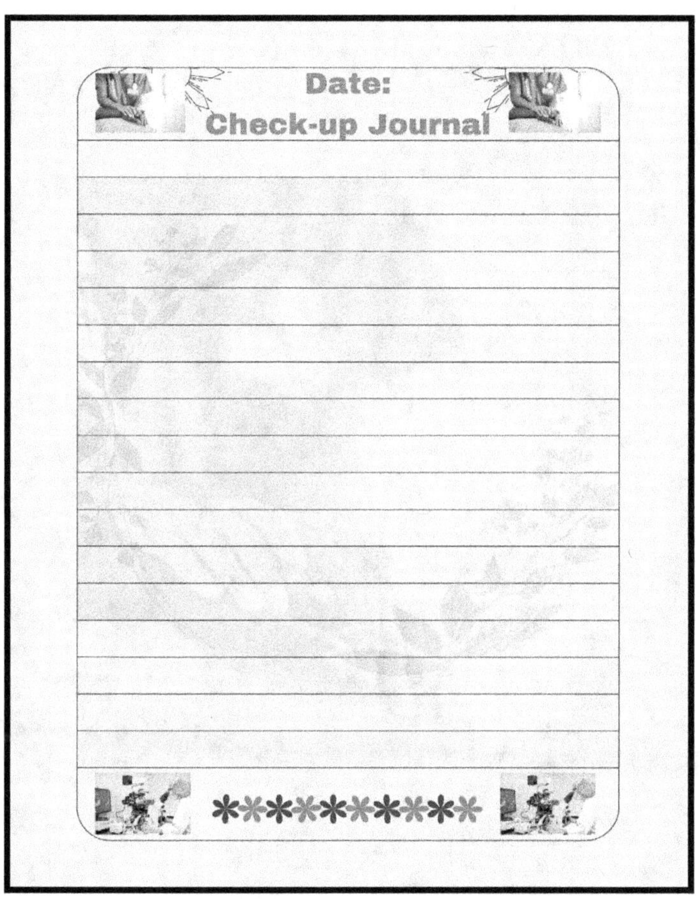

Date:
Check-up Journal